PHARMACOLOGY and TOXICOLOGY
PRACTICAL NOTEBOOK

for

Second Year Diploma in Pharmacy

(According to the new syllabus prescribed by the Pharmacy Council of India, Education Regulation 1991, implemented in the year 1993, for Diploma in Pharmacy Students)

Varun Dutt Sharma M. Pharm.   **S.K. Pandey** B. Pharm.
Principal   Sr. Lecturer

Janta Polytechnic, Jahangirabad, Bulandshahar, Uttar Pradesh

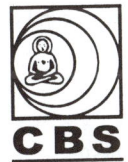

CBS

CBS Publishers & Distributors Pvt. Ltd.
New Delhi • Bengaluru • Chennai • Kochi • Kolkata • Mumbai
Hyderabad • Nagpur • Patna • Pune • Vijayawada

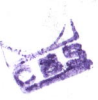
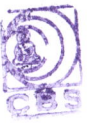

Pharmacology and
Toxicology
PRACTICAL NOTEBOOK

ISBN: 81-239-1425-3

First Edition: 2007
Reprint: 2011, 2013, 2014, 2015, 2017, 2018, 2019, 2020

Published by **Satish Kumar Jain** and produced by **Varun Jain** for
CBS Publishers & Distributors Pvt. Ltd.,
4819/XI Prahlad Street, 24 Ansari Road, Daryaganj, New Delhi - 110002
delhi@cbspd.com, cbspubs@airtelmail.in • www.cbspd.com
Ph.: 23289259, 23266861, 23266867 • Fax: 011-23243014

Corporate Office: 204 FIE, Industrial Area, Patparganj, Delhi - 110 092
Ph: 49344934 • Fax: 011-49344935
E-mail: publishing@cbspd.com • publicity@cbspd.com

Branches:
• *Bengaluru:* 2975, 17th Cross, K.R. Road, Bansankari 2nd Stage,
  Bengaluru - 70 • Ph: +91-80-26771678/79 • Fax: +91-80-26771680
  E-mail: cbsbng@gmail.com, bangalore@cbspd.com
• *Chennai:* No. 7, Subbaraya Street, Shenoy Nagar, Chennai - 600030
  Ph: +91-44-26681266, 26680620 • Fax: +91-44-42032115
  E-mail: chennai@cbspd.com
• *Kochi:* Ashana House, 39/1904, A.M. Thomas Road, Valanjambalam,
  Ernakulum, Kochi • Ph: +91-484-4059061-65
  Fax: +91-484-4059065 • E-mail: cochin@cbspd.com
• *Kolkata:* 6-B, Ground Floor, Rameshwar Shaw Road, Kolkata - 700014
  Ph: +91-33-22891126/7/8 • E-mail: kolkata@cbspd.com
• *Mumbai:* 83-C, Dr. E. Moses Road, Worli, Mumbai - 400018
  Ph: +91-9833017933, 022-24902340/41 • E-mail: mumbai@cbspd.com

Representatives:

• Hyderabad: 0-9885175004   • Nagpur: 0-9021734563
• Patna: 0-9334159340   • Pune: 0-9623451994
• Jharkhand: 0-9811541605   • Uttarakhand: 0-9716462459

Printed at:
India Binding House, Noida, UP (India)

Certificate

Student's Name _____

Class _____ Roll No. _____

This is to certify that experiments, written in the index, have been performed by the student, are satisfactory.

Grade...................   Name and signature of lab. in-charge

College stamp   Date ....

Preface

The ultimate objective of technical education is to develop relevant skill, creativity and competency among the students so as to enable them to perform the tasks effectively and efficiently later in the world of work. Practical work consists of tasks which require some manipulation of apparatus or some action.

To obtain the above aim and to reduce the writing work load to some extent to the students, this practical note book of "Pharmacology" for diploma in pharmacy second year has been written according to new syllabus as prescribed by Pharmacy council of India, education regulation 1991. This practical note book contains 17 experiments, well illustrated with graphs and experimental data to make more meaningful and guideful to the students.

Few blank pages are provided at end of this manual so that students can use these pages for writing additional experiments guided by the teachers depending on availability of reagents and infrastructure of concern laboratory.

We shall be gratefully acknowledged the comments, suggestions and criticism by respected teachers and students for improvement of future edition. We express sincere thanks to Mr Satish Kumar Jain and Mr Y.N. Arjuna, M/S CBS publishers and distributors for their cooperation, encouragement and assistance in bringing out the present form of this manual. Finally our greatest gratitude are to our colleagues and Smt. Chitra for her sincere cooperation in computer typing and setting.

Varun Dutt Sharma • S.K. Pandey

Syllabus

The first six of the following experiments will be done by the students while the remaining will be demonstrated by the teacher.

1. Effect of K^+, Ca^{++}, acetyl choline and adrenaline on frog's heart.
2. Effect or acetyl choline on rectus abdominis muscle of frog and guinea pig ileum.
3. Effect of spasmogens and relaxants on rabbit intestine.
4. Effect of local anaesthetics on rabbit cornea.
5. Effect of mydriatics and miotics on rabbit eye.
6. To study the action of strychnine on frog.
7. Effect of degitalis on frog's heart.
8. Effect of hypnotics in mice.
9. Effect of convulsants and anticonvulsants in mice or rats.
10. Test for pyrogens.
11. Taming and hypnosis potentiation effect of chlorpromazine in mice/rats.
12. Effect of diphenyl hydramine hydrochloride in experimentally produced asthma in guinea pigs.

Contents

S. No.	List of equipment for Physiology and Pharmacology Laboratry	Required No.
1.	Simple lever (Haemoglobinometer)	20
2.	Haemocytometer	10
3.	Students's organ bath	5
4.	Sherrington rotating drum	5
5.	Frog board	10
6.	Tray (dissecting)	10
7.	Frontal writing lever	15
8.	Aeration tube	20
9.	Tele thermometer	
10.	Pole climbing apparatus	1
11.	Histamine chamber	1
12.	Simple lever	15
13.	Starling heart lever	10
14.	ECG machine	—
15.	Aerator	5
16.	Histological slide	25
17.	Sphygmomanometer (B.P. apparatus)	5
18.	Stethoscope	5
19.	First aid equipment	5 sets
20.	Contraceptive device	5 sets
21.	Dissecting (surgical) instrument	20 sets
22.	Operation table (small)	2
23.	Balance for weighing small animals	1
24.	Kymograph paper	Adequate
25.	Activity cage (actophotometer)	1
26.	Analgesiometer	1
27.	Thermometer	20
28.	Distilled water still	2
29.	Plastic animal cage	10
30.	Double unit organ bath with thermostat	1
31.	Refrigerator	1
32.	Single pan balance	1
33.	Chart	Adequate
34.	Human skelton	1
35.	Anatomical specimen (Heart,brain, eye, ear, reproductive system, etc.)	1 set
36.	Electro-convulsometer	1
37.	Stop watch	10
38.	Clamp Bossheads, screw clips	Adequate
39.	Symes' Cannula	20
40.	General facilities(needles,thread Plasticiin, tubing, burners, polythene tubes, syringes, etc.	

INDEX

S. No.	Name of the experiment	Page No.	Remarks

INDEX

S. No.	Name of the experiment	Page No.	Remarks

Instructions

1. Always put on neat and clean white apron whenever you are working in the laboratory.
2. Bring always practical note book for viva and evaluation.
3. Thoroughly clean the apparatus required in the practical work.
4. Handle the animals with care. They should be treated in a human way, care being taken to avoid any injury to the handler.
5. Before any surgical procedure the animal must be anaesthetized properly.
6. The physiological solution and working solution of drug should be prepared freshly at the time of conducting experiment.
7. The stock solution of the drugs can be stored under condition specified individually.
8. Do not weigh less than 10 mg on a high quality analytical balance. For less than 10 mg of weighing of the any drug. It is advisable to prepare its solution by dilution method.
9. The practical note book should be completed in every respect and should be submitted on the same day to the teacher concerned for marking and signature.
10. Never throw waste papers and burnt match sticks in the sink, this will block the sink which may lead to over flowing. Put the waste materials in the dustbin.
11. Keep your working place neat and clean. After the work is finished the student should clean the apparatus and the other articles.
12. The water taps and gas taps should be tightly closed after the work is over.
13. Never take and use any chemical or reagents prior taking permission from the teacher or the lab. technician.
14. Always be in college uniform and maintain strict discipline.
15. Electrical switches should be put off before leaving the laboratory.

USEFUL TABLES

Physiological salt solutions

Ingredients	Concentration in gram per litre				
	Frog ringer	Ringer locke	Krebs	Tyrode	Dejalon
NaCl	6.5	0.9	6.9	8.0	9.0
KCl	0.14	0.42	0.35	0.2	0.42
$CaCl_2$	0.12	0.24	0.28	0.2	0.06
$MgSO_47H_2O$	-	-	0.28	-	-
$NaH_2PO_42H_2O$	0.05	-	-	0.1	-
KH_2PO_4	-	-	0.16	-	-
$NaHCO_3$	0.4	0.5	2.1	1.0	0.5
Glucose	1.5	1.0	2.1	1.0	0.5
$MgCl_2$	-	-	-	0.1	-
Distilled water	1000 ml	1000 ml	1000 ml	1000 ml	1000 ml

Anaesthetic agents used in laboratory animals

General anaesthetics are those drugs which produce reversible loss of consciousness, skeletal muscle relaxation and loss of memory.

Drug	Concentration	Animal	Dose per kg	Route
Urethane	25%	Rabbit	0.5–1.75 g	IV
	50%	Guinea pig	1.5 g	IP
	25%	Rat	1.25–1.75 g	IM or SC
Pentobarbitone	6%	Rabbit	50–60 mg	IV
	1%	Guinea pig	30–50 mg	IP
	0.6%	Rat, mouse	30–60 mg	IP

Urethane: It is freely soluble in water.
It is suitable for rats and rabbits.
Anaesthesia lasts for three to four hours.

Pentobarbitone: It is generally used in 6% solution and is dissolved in 10% alcohol.
Induction of anaesthesia is rapid and lasts four half an hour to one hour.

Experimental animals

Animal	Rectal temp. in °C	Pulse rate per minute	Respiratory rate per minute	Gestation period	Adult weight	Average life span	Age of mating
Mouse	37.4	600	163	19 days	20–40 gm	18 months–2 years	45–60 days
Rat	37.5	300	210	21 days	150–250 gm	2–3 Years	2.5–3 months
Rabbit	38.7	135	55	28 days	1.5–5 kg	4–6 Years	6–7 months
Guinea pig	38.6	150	80	66 days	450–800 gm	3–5 Years	3 months

Observation table

Sl. No.	Drug used	Heart rate	Amplitude of contraction in mm	Response of myocardial muscles of heart
1.	No drug	——	—— mm	Normal
2.	Acetylcholine	——	—— mm	Decrease
3.	KCl	——	—— mm	Decrease
4.	Adrenaline	——	—— mm	Increase
5.	$CaCl_2$	——	—— mm	Increase

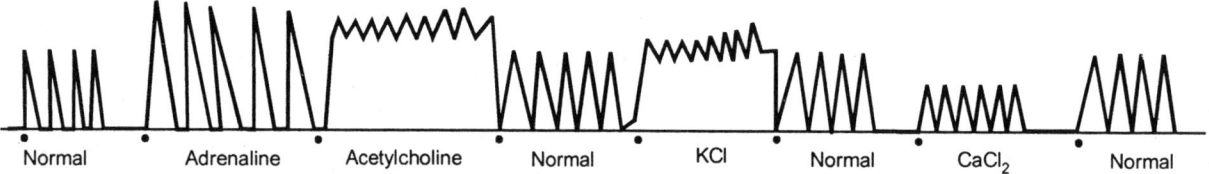

Normal   Adrenaline   Acetylcholine   Normal   KCl   Normal $CaCl_2$ Normal

Effect of various drugs on perfused frog's heart

Experiment 1

OBJECT

To study the effect of K^+, Ca^{++}, acetylcholine and adrenaline on perfused frog's heart .

Requirements

Recording drum, Sterling's heart lever, venous cannula and thread.

Chemicals

Calcium chloride, acetylcholine, KCl, $CaCl_2$, frog's ringer solution, etc.

Principle

Acetylcholine

It is parasympathomimetic drug. Muscarinic receptor is found in heart. In the heart acetylcholine causes activation of potassium ion channel, account for negative chronotropism (decrease heart rate) and negative inotropism (decrease force of contraction). Thus, the heart is inhibited. In perfused frog heart preparations stoppage of the heart is seen on upper side, while in isolated preparation it stops in diastolic condition.

Adrenaline

It is sympathomimetic having mixed agonists action. It produces increase in heart rate (positive chronotropic effect) and force of contraction (positive inotropic effect). Thus, adrenaline produces direct excitatory action on myocardial muscles mediated through ß receptors present in the heart.

Calcium Chloride

In lower doses it increases heart rate and force of contraction but in high doses it inhibits the heart in systole characterized by straight line on upper side in isolated heart and on lower side in perfused frog heart.

Potassium chloride

It has also inhibitory effect on heart. In perfused frog heart preparation, it stops in systole while in isolated preparation, it stops in diastole.

Procedure

Take a pithed healthy frog in dissecting tray. Start dissection on ventral surface to expose the heart. While dissecting, abdominal aorta should be intact. Remove the pericardium carefully. Tie the branch of the aorta with a thread. The venous cannula is inserted into inferior vena cava by making an incision followed by constant washing with frog's ringer solution. Cut off a branch of the aorta and adjust the flow of frog's ringer solution. Pass a hook through apex of ventricle, connect it with thread to starlings heart lever. Observe the normal force and frequency of heart. Inject acetyl choline (10 µg) through the rubber tube. Start drum and record response for One minute. Stop drum and let the response to be normal again. Repeat the above procedure for KCl (2.5 mg), adrenaline (10 µg), $CaCl_2$ (2.5 mg) followed by 5 mg respectively. Record the graph, label it and then fix the graph with alcoholic reginous solution.

Result

Acetylcholine	——	Excitatory action on heart muscles/Inhibitory action on heart muscles
KCl	——	Excitatory action on heart muscles/Inhibitory action on heart muscles
Adrenaline	——	Excitatory action on heart muscles/Inhibitory action on heart muscles
CaCl$_2$	——	Excitatory action on heart muscles/Inhibitory action on heart muscles

Reagents and drugs

Frog's Ringer solution: It should be freshly prepared.

Acetylcholine (100 µg/ml): It is hygroscopic and unstable in aqueous solution. So It should be prepared freshly at the time of experiment. Its stock solution is made in 5% NaH_2PO_4. Weigh 10 mg of acetylcholine and dissolve in 10 ml of 5% NaH_2PO_4 solution. For making working stock solution (10 µg), take 0.1 ml of above stock solution and diluted 10 ml with distilled water.

Adrenaline solution (100 µg/ml): It is available as hydrochloride or hydrogen tartrate. The stock solution is prepared in 1% ascorbic acid to decrease oxidation.

Weigh 10 mg adrenaline and dissolve in 10 ml 1% ascorbic acid solution. Take 0.5 ml of above stock solution and dilute to 5 ml with distilled water. This will give 100 µg/ml of adrenaline solution.

KCl (10 mg/ml): Dissolve 1 g of potassium chloride in 100 ml of distilled water.

CaCl$_2$ (10 mg/ml): Dissolve 1 gram of calcium chloride (anhydrous) in 100 ml of distilled water.

Observation table

S. No.	Drug used	Heart rate	Amplitude of contraction in mm	Response of myocardial muscles of heart
1.	No drug	——	—— mm	Normal
2.	Acetyl choline	——	—— mm	Decrease
3.	KCl	——	—— mm	Decrease
4.	Adrenaline	——	—— mm	Increase
5.	CaCl$_2$	——	—— mm	Increase

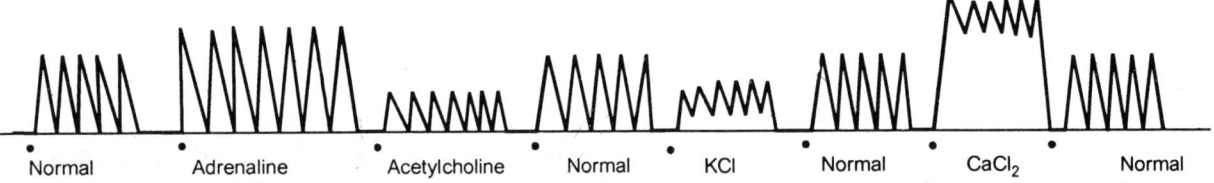

Effect of various drugs on isolated frog heart

Experiment 2

OBJECT

To study the effect of K^+, Ca^{++}, acetylcholine and adrenaline on frog's isolated heart.

Requirements

Recording drum, Sterling's heart lever, Syme's Cannula and thread.

Chemicals

Calcium Chloride, Acetylcholine, KCl, $CaCl_2$, frog's ringer solution, etc.

Principle

Acetylcholine: It is parasympathomimetic drug. Muscarinic receptor is found in heart. In the heart acetylcholine causes activation of potassium ion channel, account for negative chronotropism (Decrease heart rate) and negative inotropism (Decrease force of contraction). Thus, the heart is inhibited. In perfused frog heart preparations stoppage of the heart is seen on upper side, while in isolated preparation it stops in diastolic condition.

Adrenaline

It is sympathomimetic having mixed agonists action. It produces increase in heart rate (positive chronotropic effect) and force of contraction (positive inotropic effect). Thus, adrenaline produces direct excitatory action on myocardial muscles mediated through β receptors present in the heart.

Calcium Chloride

In lower doses it increases heart rate and force of contraction but in high doses it inhibits the heart in systole characterized by straight line on upper side in isolated heart and on lower side in perfused frog heart.

Potassium chloride

It has also inhibitory effect on heart. In perfused frog heart preparation, it stops in systole while in isolated preparation, it stops in diastole.

Procedure

Take a pithed healthy frog in dissecting tray. Start dissection on ventral surface to expose the heart while dissecting, abdominal aorta should be intact. Remove the pericardium carefully. Insert Syme's cannula into inferior vena cava and isolate the heart outside the body. Place isolated heart in heart chamber and start perfusion ringers solution at about 20 drops per minute. Pass the hook through apex of ventricle, Connect it with thread to starlings heart lever. Observe the normal force and frequency of heart.

Inject acetylcholine (10 μg) into Syme's cannula. Start drum and record response for one minute. Stop drum and let the response to be normal again. Repeat the above procedure for KCl (2.5 mg), adrenaline (10 μg), $CaCl_2$ 2.5 mg followed by 5 mg respectively. Record the graph, label it and then fix the kymograph paper containing responses of various drug with alcoholic reginous solution.

Result

Acetylcholine	——	Excitatory action on heart muscles/Inhibitory action on heart muscles
KCl	——	Excitatory action on heart muscles/Inhibitory action on heart muscles
Adrenaline	——	Excitatory action on heart muscles/Inhibitory action on heart muscles
$CaCl_2$	——	Excitatory action on heart muscles/Inhibitory action on heart muscles

Drug	Perfused heart	Isolated heart
Acetylcholine	Stoppage of heart preparation on upper side (systole)	Stoppage of heart on down side (diastolic condition)
KCl	Stoppage of heart preparation on upper side (systole)	Stoppage of heart on down side (diastolic condition)
Adrenaline	Stoppage of heart preparation on upper side (systole)	Stoppage of heart on down side (diastolic condition)
$CaCl_2$ (high dose 1% or more)	Inhibition of the heart response on lower side	Inhibition of the heart response on upper side

Observation table

S. No.	Dose of actylcholine	Amplitude of response in mm
1.	(.05 ml) 5 µg	
2.	(0.1 ml) 10 µg	
3.	(0.2 ml) 20 µg	
4.	(0.4 ml) 40 µg	

Actylcholine (100 µg/ml)–Weigh 10 mg of actylcholine and dissolve in 10 ml 5% NaH_2PO_4. For making working actylcholine solution, take 1 ml of above stock solution and is diluted to 10 ml with distilled water.

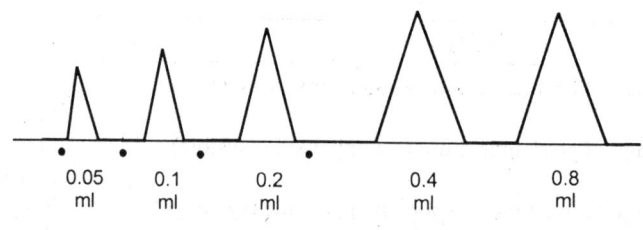

| 0.05 ml | 0.1 ml | 0.2 ml | 0.4 ml | 0.8 ml |

Drug—Acetylcholine

Experiment 3

OBJECT

To study the effect of acetylcholine on rectus abdominis muscles of frog .

Requirements

Organ bath, recording drum, frontal writing lever, thread and syringe with needle.

Chemicals

Frog's ringer solution, acetylcholine (100 μg per ml), etc.

Principle

Acetylcholine is parasympathomimetic or cholinergic drug, is synthesized inside the nerve fibre by the combination of choline with acetyl group obtained from acetyl co-enzyme–A in presence of enzyme acetylase. The released acetylcholine acts on postsynaptic receptors, i.e. muscarinic or nicotinic receptors. Nicotinic receptors are found in autonomic ganglia, skeletal muscles and certain sites of central nervous system. The action of acetylcholine is terminated by hydrolysis through the enzyme cholinesterase. Nicotinic receptors found in skeletal muscles are responsible for the end plate potential and neuromuscular transmission. Rectus abdominis muscle is a skeletal muscle and actylcholine causes contraction through nicotinic receptor. d-Tubocurarine is nicotinic receptor blocker which reduces the response of acetylcholine.

Procedure

Take the pithed frog in dissecting tray. Incise the skin of abdomen. Dissect the rectus abdominis muscle from pelvic region to thorax part of the frog. Tie threads on both ends of the muscle and transfer it in inner organ bath containing frog's ringer solution at room temperature. The one end of the thread is attached to aeration tube and other end to lever. Stabilize the isolated muscle for 30–45 minutes. Then add minimum dose of actylcholine in a bath by means of syringe, start drum and record the effect on a kymograph for 1.5 minute. Stop drum and wash the preparation. Adjust the lever at base line. Repeat the procedure by adding actylcholine at dose 10 μg, 20 μg, 40 μg and record the responses. Fix the graph.

Result

Acetylcholine produces contraction of rectus abdominis muscles (Skeletal muscle) of frog.

Observation table

S. No.	Drug dose	Amplitude of response	Response
1.	No drug	——————— cm	Normal
2.	Acetylcholine (0.05 ml)	——————— cm	Increase
3.	Acetylcholine (0.1 ml)	——————— cm	Increase
4.	Acetylcholine (0.2 ml)	——————— cm	Increase
5.	Acetylcholine (0.4 ml)	——————— cm	Increase

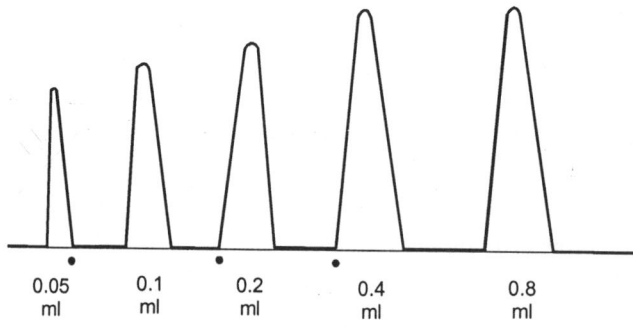

Drug—Acetylcholine

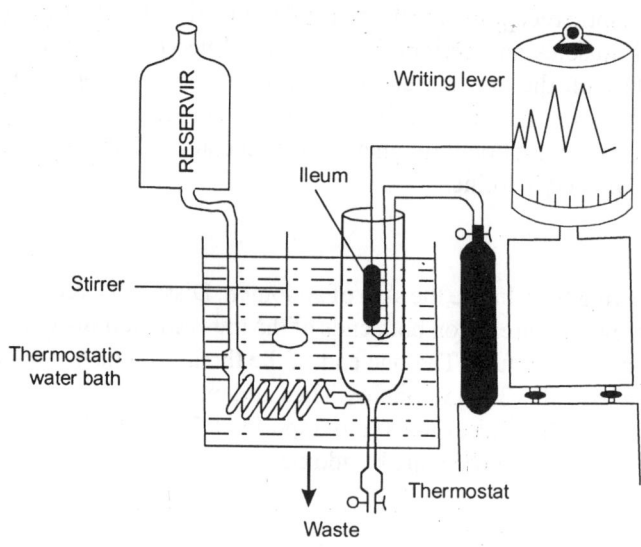

Assembly for isolated tissue.

Experiment 4

OBJECT

To study the effect of acetylcholine on guinea pig ileum.

Requirements

Organ bath, recording drum, frontal writing lever, thread, etc.

Chemicals

Acetylcholine (100 µg/ml) and Tyrode solution.

Principle

Acetylcholine is parasympathomimetic or cholinergic drug and each synthesized inside the nerve fibre by the combination of choline with acetyl group obtained from acetyl co-enzyme–A in the presence of enzyme acetylase. The released acetylcholine acts on postsynaptic receptors muscarinic or nicotinic receptor. Muscarinic receptors are found in all type of smooth muscles, heart and exocrine glands. Acetylcholine causes increase in tone, motility and peristalsis. Isolated guinea pig ileum (smooth muscle) shows normal pendular peristalsis under the influence of acetylcholine.

Procedure

Healthy guinea pig is killed by stunning (blow on the head). Take guinea pig in dissecting tray. Abdomen is opened through a mid line incision. Locate the ileum near the ileocaecal junction. Cut a 10 cm piece of ileum. Gently remove mesenteries. Lumen of ileum is washed and cleaned by warm tyrode solution. Tie the thread on both ends. One end of ileum is tied to aeration tube hook and other to the lever. Inner organ bath is filled with tyrode solution. Outer organ bath is thermostatically controlled at 37° C.

Start the drum and sketch the base line on smoked kymograph paper. Stabilize the tissue for sufficient time and take the normal response of the tissue. Record responses of acetylcholine at doses of 0.05 ml, 0.1 ml, 0.2 ml and 0.4 ml, etc. for one minute respectively. Stop the drum and wash the preparation at each dose addition. At each washing fresh tyrode solution is filled in inner organ bath. Fix the graph by reginous solution.

Result

Acetylcholine increases the contraction of ileum of guinea pig.

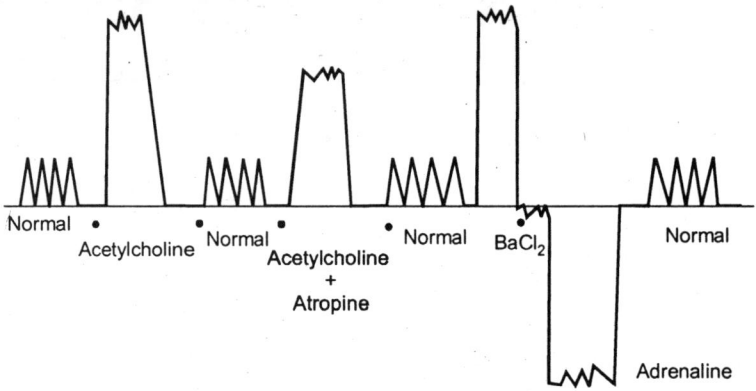

Effect of drugs on rabbit intestine

Experiment 5

OBJECT

To study the effect of spasmogens and relaxants on rabbit intestine.

Requirements

Organ bath, recording drum, frontal writing lever and thread.

Chemicals

Acetylcholine, atropine, $BaCl_2$, adrenaline and mammalian ringer solution.

Principle

Spasmogens are those drugs which bring about spasm, i.e. sudden involuntary contraction of muscles. The cholinergic drugs like acetylcholine, carbachol are spasmodic agents, produce increase in motility, amplitude and tone of muscles. This action is mediated through muscarinic receptor. Barium chloride causes increase in tone by direct effect. Directly acting spasmogenic drugs are ergot, ADH and $BaCl_2$. Action of $BaCl_2$ cannot be block while action of acetylcholine can be blocked by atropine (antimuscarinic action). Spasmogens have got therapeutic value in treatment of paralytic ileus and atony of bladder.

Relaxants are those drugs which induce relaxation. They are also called antispasmodics. Sympathomimetics like adrenaline and noradrenaline relax the rabbit intestine. Relaxation of smooth muscle also caused by potassium ions. Higher dose of caffeine also causes relaxation of gut. Relaxants are therapeutically used as a pre-anaesthetics agents.

Procedure

Fill the inner organ bath with mammalian ringer solution. Outer organ bath is thermostatically controlled at 37.5° C. A rabbit is killed by head blow (Stunning) method and bled to death. The animal is dissected out, the abdominal organs are exposed to isolate a piece of intestine (5–8 cm) in length. Remove adhering blood vessels and mesentery and cleaned the lumen of intestine. Ligate the both ends with thread. Tie one end to the aeration tube and suspend it in bath containing mammalian ringer solution. The other end is connected to lever for tracing. Normal response is recorded on rotating drum.

Start the drum and add acetylcholine (0.1 ml) to the bath and record the effect for one minute. Stop the drum. Wash the preparation with ringer solution and allow to the muscle to relax. Washings of tissue should be done several times to remove the effect of previous drugs. Similarly repeat procedure for barium chloride (2 ml) and adrenaline (0.1 ml). The combine effect of acetylcholine (0.1 ml) and atropine (0.1 ml) is recorded in similar manner. Fix the graph.

Result

Acetylcholine and barium chloride being spasmogenic drugs increase the tone and force of contraction while adrenaline causes relaxation. Atropine being anti-muscarinic agent antagonizes the action of acetylcholine.

Reagents

Mammalian Ringer solution

Sodium chloride	—9 g
Potassium chloride	—0.42 g
Calcium chloride	—0.24 g
Sodium bicarbonate	—0.5 g
Glucose	—1 g
Magnesium chloride	—0.1 g
Sodium dihydrogen phosphate	—0.1 g
Distilled water	—1000 ml

Acetyl choline (100 μg/ml)

Weigh 10 mg of acetyl choline and dissolve in 10 ml of 5% sodium dihydrogen phosphate solution. For making working acetyl choline solution, take 1 ml of above stock solution and is diluted to 10 ml with distilled water.

Adrenaline (100 μg/ml)

Weigh accurately 10 mg of adrenaline and dissolve in 10 ml of 1% ascorbic acid solution. Take 0.5 ml of the above stock solution and is diluted to 5 ml with distilled water.

Barium chloride (1 mg per ml)

Weigh accurately 10 mg and dissolve in 10 ml of distilled water.

Atropine solution (50 μg/ml)

Weigh accurately 10 mg and dissolve in 10 ml of distilled water. Take 0.5 ml of the above stock solution and is diluted to 10 ml with distilled water.

Observation table

| Time in minute | Corneal reflex | |
	right eye as control	left eye treated with 1% xylocaine solution
1.	Positive	
2.	Positive	
3.	Positive	
4.	Positive	
5.	Positive	
6.	Positive	
7.	Positive	
8.	Positive	
9.	Positive	
10.	Positive	
11.	Positive	
12.	Positive	
13.	Positive	
14.	Positive	
15.	Positive	

Drug	Trade name	Name of Company
Xylocaine 1%	Xylocaine	ASTRA ZENECA

Experiment 6

OBJECT

To study the effect of local anaesthetics on rabbit cornea.

Requirements

Rabbits, Rabbit holder, dropper, etc.

Drug

1% xylocaine.

Principle

Local anaesthetics are those drugs which cause reversible loss of the nerve conduction and hence loss of sensory perception of pain when applied locally. An ideal local anaesthetics have the following characteristics.

1. They should not cause irritation.
2. Onset of action should be quick.
3. Duration of action should be sufficient.
4. They should be free from systemic toxicity.
5. They should be stable.

Local anaesthetics produce their effect by inhibiting the permeability of sodium ions and hence prevent depolarization. They displace calcium ions from their binding site. Thus they reduce the rate and rise of action potential and block the conduction of impulses. Lignocaine is used as a surface, infiltration, nerve block and spinal anaesthesia. This experiment can detect activity of lignocaine as surface anaesthetic agent. Absence of corneal reflex is indicative of local anaesthetic activity.

Procedure

Select healthy rabbit and place in holder box. Cut off the eye lashes of the rabbit at least 24 hours before starting experiment since eye lashes interfere with corneal reflex. Keep right eye as control and treat left eye for conducting experiment. Observe the corneal reflexes in both eyes with a wick of cotton. To test corneal reflex, approach the animal from its side and then touch the cornea with wick of cotton. If the hand is brought from front, the animal visualizes the hands and closes the eye. Put 2-3 drops of xylocaine (1%) in left eye and examine the corneal reflex after every one minute. Report the on set and duration of action of xylocaine. The loss of corneal reflex is the indicative of the onset of action of the drug. Positive corneal reflex is the indication of the recovery of corneal sensation.

Result

On set of action ....minutes
Duration of action ....minutes

Observations

Drug	Pupil size	Light reflex	Corneal reflex
Pilocarpine	Decrease	Present	Present
Physostigmine	Decrease	Present	Present
Ephedrine	Increase	Present	Present
Atropine	Increase	Absent	Present
Phenylephrine	Increase	Present	Present

Pilocarpine

Time in minutes	Pupil size in mm		Corneal reflex		Light reflex	
	Control eye	Test eye	Control eye	Test eye	Control eye	Test eye
0 minute (no drug)	-	-	-	-	-	-
10 minutes	-	-	-	-	-	-
20 minutes	-	-	-	-	-	-
30 minutes	-	-	-	-	-	-
40 minutes	-	-	-	-	-	-

Physostigmine

Time in minutes	Pupil size in mm		Corneal reflex		Light reflex	
	Control eye	Test eye	Control eye	Test eye	Control eye	Test eye
0 minute (no drug)	-	-	-	-	-	-
10 minutes	-	-	-	-	-	-
20 minutes	-	-	-	-	-	-
30 minutes	-	-	-	-	-	-
40 minutes	-	-	-	-	-	-

Ephedrine

Time in minutes	Pupil size in mm		Corneal reflex		Light reflex	
	Control eye	Test eye	Control eye	Test eye	Control eye	Test eye
0 minute (no drug)	-	-	-	-	-	-
10 minutes	-	-	-	-	-	-
20 minutes	-	-	-	-	-	-
30 minutes	-	-	-	-	-	-
40 minutes	-	-	-	-	-	-

Experiment 7

OBJECT

To study the effect of mydriatics and miotics on rabbit eye.

Requirements

Rabbit, dropper, rabbit holder, scale, scissor, etc.

Chemicals

Pilocarpine 4%, physostigmine 0.5–1%, phenylephrine 10%, atropine 0.1% and ephedrine 5%.

Principle

Mydriatics are those which dilate the pupil and miotics are those which constrict the pupil. Mydriasis is produced by parasympatholytic agents example atropine, homatropine; sympathomimetics, e.g. adrenaline, phenylephrine, ephedrine, and local anaesthetic, e.g. cocaine.

Miosis are produced by parasympathomimetic drugs, e.g. pilocarpine, physostigmine, etc. Pupil has to muscles, i.e. the circular muscle and the radial muscle. Miosis is produced by contraction of the circular muscle which is stimulated by parasympathomimetics such as physostigmine. Mydriasis or dilatation of the pupil is produced by either contraction of the radial muscle or paralysis of circular muscle. Thus, sympathomimetics (phenylephrine) and parasympatholytics (atropine and homatropine) both produce dilatation of pupil.

Procedure

Take five rabbits, one rabbit for each drug. Cut off the eye lashes of the each rabbit. Keep left eye as control and instill 2 to 3 drops of drugs in right eye. After 10 minutes of instillation of a drug. Observe pupil size, corneal reflex and light reflex at every 10 minutes of the interval. Corneal reflex is observed by touching cotton wicks from the side of the rabbit. The blinking response is obtained. The pupil size is determined by a transparent scale. Light reflex is elicited by throwing light from pen torch on eye and watch for constriction of the pupil.

Atropine

Time in minutes	Pupil size in mm		Corneal reflex		Light reflex	
	Control eye	Test eye	Control eye	Test eye	Control eye	Test eye
0 minute (no drug)	-	-	-	-	-	-
10 minutes	-	-	-	-	-	-
20 minutes	-	-	-	-	-	-
30 minutes	-	-	-	-	-	-
40 minutes	-	-	-	-	-	-

Phenylephrine

Time in minutes	Pupil size in mm		Corneal reflex		Light reflex	
	Control eye	Test eye	Control eye	Test eye	Control eye	Test eye
0 minute (no drug)	-	-	-	-	-	-
10 minutes	-	-	-	-	-	-
20 minutes	-	-	-	-	-	-
30 minutes	-	-	-	-	-	-
40 minutes	-	-	-	-	-	-

Note: Keep left eye as control and test eye for instillation of the drug.

Drug	Trade Name	Name of company
Atropine	Atro Eye Drops	INTAS
Ephedrine	Endrine Eye Drops	WYETH LEDERLE
Phenylephrine HCl	Fenox Drops	KNOLL
Pilocarpine (4%)	Pilocar Drops	FDC

Result

Mydriatics (dilatation of the pupil): Atropine, ephedrine, phenylephrine.
Miotics (constriction of the pupil): Pilocarpine, physostigmine.

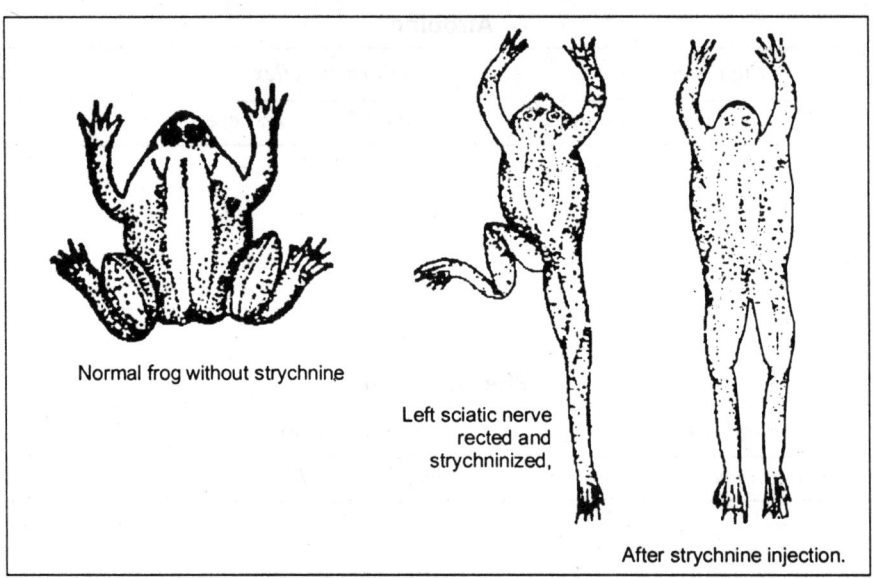

Normal frog without strychnine

Left sciatic nerve
rected and
strychninized,

After strychnine injection.

Strychnine effect on frog: N. Normal frog without strychnine A. Left sciatic nerve rected and strychninized, B. After strychnine injection.

Experiment 8

OBJECT

To study the action of strychnine on frog.

Requirements

Syringe with needle.

Chemical

Strychnine

Prepare 100 μg/per ml of strychnine. Weigh accurately 10 mg of strychnine in 10 ml distilled water. Take 1 ml of above stock solution and is diluted to 10 ml with distilled water. This will give 100 μg/per ml of strychnine.

Principle

Strychnine is an alkaloid obtained from the seed of *Strychnus nuxvomica*. It is an analeptic drug and produces its effect through inhibition of glycine of CNS (brain and spinal cord). If used in excess It may give rise to tonic type of convulsions which involve both the flexor and extensor group of muscles. Its poisoning is characterized by tonic convulsions, lock jaw and bending of the body.

Procedure

Take a healthy frog and inject strychnine solution intramuscularly. The dose should be given slightly in excess. Record the appearance of convulsions. The jerking movement of the lower limb is indicative of the initiation of the convulsive effect. Report the on set of action after giving the injection and mortality time.

Result

Strychnine causes tonic type of convulsions, lock jaw and arc like body.

On set of action - ……………………..

Mortality time - ………………………

	Size of the heart	Extent of contraction
Normal		
Digitalised Heart		
Diseased heart prior to failure		
Failing Heart		
After digitalisation		

Digitalis action: 1. Normal and digitalized heart.
2. Diseased heart and digitalisation.

Experiment 9

OBJECT

To study the effect of digitalis on frog's heart.

Requirements

Starlings heart lever, venous cannula, recording drum, kymograph paper, stand and thread.

Chemicals

Digoxin solution (100 µg/per ml): Weigh 10 mg of digoxin and dissolve in 10 ml distilled water. Take 1 ml of above stock solution and is diluted to 10 ml with distilled water.
1. Physiological salt solution.
    (a) Frog's ringer solution.
    (b) Frog's ringer solution without calcium chloride.
2. Calcium chloride solution 4%.

Principle

Digitalis being cardiotonic, discovered by William withering in 1976, has been therapeutically used in treatment of congestive cardiac failure (CCF). It inhibits a $Na^+ K^+$ ATP ase and there by increases inflex of sodium ions. This causes increase in calcium ions intracellularly and hence an increase in force of contraction of heart. Due to increase in the end diastolic volume and decrease in the force of contraction of the heart of CCF patient, the size of the heart is increased. When digitalis is given to the CCF patient, there is increase in force of contraction of the heart. Due to decrease in the end diastolic volume, the size of the heart is also decreased. Digitalis increases the utilization of the energy production. Calcium ions play an important role in myocardial muscle contractility. When the heart is perfused with frog's ringer solution without calcium chloride, there is decrease in the force of contraction of the heart. But when this physiological solution is replaced with normal frog's ringer solution containing calcium chloride followed by gradual adding the dose of digoxin, there is increase in performance of the heart contractility. It is evident that digitalis and calcium ions both act synergistically.

Procedure

Take a pithed healthy frog in a dissecting tray. Start dissection on ventral surface to expose the heart. While dissecting, the abdominal aorta should be intact. Remove the pericardium carefully. Tie the branch of aorta with a thread. The venous cannula is inserted into inferior vena cava by making an incision followed by constant washing with frog's ringer solution. Cut off the branch of the aorta and adjust the flow of frog's ringer solution (15–20 drops per minute). Pass a hook through apex of ventricle, connect it with thread to starlings heart lever. Observe the normal extent of contraction of the cardiac muscles and the size of the heart.

Inject digoxin 0.1 ml through rubber tube. Start drum and record response for one minute. Stop drum and let the response to be normal again. Repeat the above procedure for 0.2 ml and 0.4 ml of digoxin replace the normal ringer solution with ringer solution without calcium chloride and record the response of the heart. Administer digoxin 0.1 ml and 0.2 ml along with calcium chloride of dos e 0.1 ml and 0.2 ml respectively. Record and observe the response again. Immediate improvement of the cardiac performance is seen.

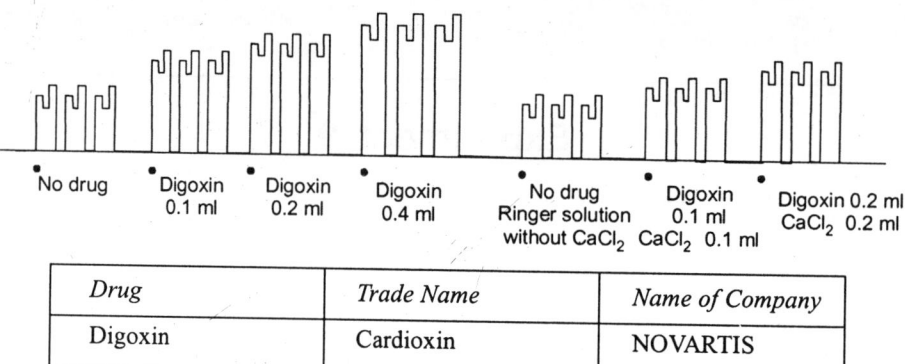

Drug	Trade Name	Name of Company
Digoxin	Cardioxin	NOVARTIS

S. No.	Physiological salt solution	Drug	Extent of contraction	Size of the heart
1.	Ringer solution	No drug	Normal	Normal
2.	Ringer solution	Digoxin (0.1 ml)	Increase	Decrease
3.	Ringer solution	Digoxin (0.2 ml)	Increase	Decrease
4.	Ringer solution	Digoxin (0.4 ml)	Increase	Decrease
5.	Ringer solution without calcium chloride	No drug	Decrease	No significant effect
6.	Ringer solution without calcium chloride	Digoxin (0.1 ml) + $CaCl_2$ (0.1 ml) of 4%	Increase	Decrease
7.	Ringer solution without calcium chloride	Digoxin (0.2 ml) + $CaCl_2$ (0.2 ml) of 4%	Increase	Decrease

Result

Digitalis along with calcium ions have synergistic effect on contractility power of the heart muscles. Depression of the contractility of the cardiac muscles can overcome by digitalis and calcium chloride administration. Digitalis decreases the size of the heart.

Drug	Trade Name	Name of company
Phenobarbitone	Gardenal injection	NICHOLAS
Diazepam	Calmpose injection	RANBAXY

Experiment 10

OBJECT

To study the effect of hypnotics in mice.

Chemicals

Phenobarbitone 15 mg per kg, diazepam 4 mg per kg.

Principle

Hypnotics are those drugs which induce sleep. Most sedatives in larger doses produces hypnosis. Sleep is temporary interruption of awakefullness. It is very essential in life. A normal sleep has two phases one non rapid eye movement (NREM) and second rapid eye movement (REM). Although REM sleep is disturbing phase but it is concern with repair of mental fatigue. Lack of this phase may cause irritation and other psychological disturbance. Hypnotics are therapeutically used in treatment of insomnia. An ideal hypnotics should be nontoxic non-addictive and free from hang over effect.

Barbiturates and benzodiazepines are two important group of hypnotics which are widely used in clinical practices. Depending on duration of action barbiturates are further divided in to long acting, intermediate and short acting. Benzodiazepines have higher therapeutic index, e.g. dizepam, oxazepam, lorazepam, etc. They induce sleep which is almost identical to normal sleep as the REM component is not suppressed while in barbiturates it is depressed.

Procedure

Take three healthy mice of either sex. They are marked one, two and three respectively. Inject one ml of saline solution intraperitonealy to the mouse no. 1. Mouse no. 2 and 3 are administered phenobarbitone 15 mg per kg body weight and diazepam 4 mg per kg body weight respectively and report the on set of action and duration of action of phenobarbitone and diazepam. Loss of righting reflex of the mice is the indicative of the initiation of the hypnosis effect of the drugs.

Righting reflex: Restoration of the normal posture by the animal which is drop from height on soft surface of the table is termed as righting reflex.

The saline treated mouse is kept as control.

Result

On set of hypnosis action.
  (a) Phenobarbitone sodium ....
  (b) Diazepam ....
      Duration of action

Observation table

Rat No.	Drug	Dose in mg/kg	Convulsion	
			jerking movement of animal	mortality/ recovery
02	Pentylene tetrazole	80 mg/kg	....	
02	Trimethadione + pentyletetrazole	400 mg/kg + 80 mg/kg	....	
02	Diazepam + Pentylenetetrazole	4 mg/kg + 80 mg/kg	....	

Experiment 11

OBJECT

To study the effect of convulsants and anticonvulsants in mice or rats.

Chemicals

Pentylene tetrazole (Leptazole).
Dose–80 mg per kg subcuteneously.
Trimethadione–400 mg per kg orally.
Diazepam–4 mg per kg intraperitoneally.

Theory

Convulsion can be produced in mice by injecting analeptics like strychnine (1 mg per kg) or pentylenetetrazol (Leptazol). Drugs that are effective in electrically induced seizures are found to be beneficial in grand-mal epilepsy where as those effective in chemically induced seizures are found to be useful in petit-mal epilepsy.

Anticonvulsants are antiepileptic agents. Antiepileptic drugs cause normalization of seizure foci, prevention of post-tetanic potential, potentiation of pre- or postsynaptic inhibition and prolongation of the refractory period. Trimethodione blocks chemically induced seizures and is used in treatment of petitmal epilepsy. It increases threshold of excitability in thalamus and depresses polysynaptic transmission. Dizepam also prevents chemically induced seizures and suppress spread of seizures. It stimulates the GABA receptors.

Procedure

Select six healthy rats or mice. Two of them are fed trimethadione (400 mg per kg) orally. After one hour both mice/rats are injected pentylene tetrazole intraperitoneally. Another two mice/rats are injected diazepam (4 mg per kg) intraperitoneally. After half an hour all the rest four mice/rats are injected pentylene tetrazole intraperitoneally. Record the presence or absence of convulsions. Abolition of both tonic and clonic seizures in 50% of animals is criteria for anticonvulsant activity of drugs.

Result

Trimethadione and diazepam are anticonvulsant drugs because they protect convulsive seizures of rats/mice where as pentylenetetrazole is convulsive drug.

Experiment 12

OBJECT

To carry out test for pyrogen IP edition 1996 (preliminary test).

Requirements

Syringes, needles, glassware, rabbit, rabbit holder, oven, telethermameter, etc.

Chemicals

saline solution (pyrogen free) and test solution.

Principle

The test is performed for those aqueous parenteral preparations whose pyrogen test is specified in Indian pharmacopoeia (1996 edition) under their individual monograph. The test involves measurements of the rise in body temperature of rabbits following the intravenous injection of a sterile solution of substances being examined.

Dose

Volume of injection is not less than 0.5 ml per kg and not more than 10 ml per kg body weight.

Test animal

Take healthy rabbit of either sex, weighing not less than 1.5 kg, fed on complete and balanced diet and not showing loss of body weight during the week preceding the test. Keep the animal in an area of uniform temperature ($\pm 2°$) and humidity free from disturbances likely to excite them.

Materials

All glassware, syringes and needles must be thoroughly washed with water for injection and heated in a hot air oven at 250° C for thirty minutes or at 200° C for one hour to assure their sterility and free from pyrogen. The animals are put in to retaining boxes one hour before the test and remain in them throughout the test. The retaining box should be such that the animal may move freely. With hold food from the animals over night and until the test is completed. Withhold water during the test.

Recording the temperature

Insert the clinical thermometer or probes of telethermometer in to the rectum of the test rabbit to a depth of about 5 cm. The depth of insertion is constant for any one rabbit in any one test.

Preliminary test

Sham test: If animals are used for the first time in the pyrogen tests or have not been used during the two previous weeks, inject 10 ml per kg body wt. of a pyrogen free saline solution intravenously warmed at about 38.5° C. Record the temperature of the animals beginning at least 90 minutes before injection and continuing for three hours after injection of the solution. Any animal showing temperature variation of 0.6° C or more must not be used in the main test.

Result

The selected rabbits should be marked and kept for main test.

Observation table

Rabbit I			Rabbit II			Rabbit III			Summed up responses of three rabbits
Temperature in °C			Temperature °C			Temperature in °C			
Before injection	After injection	Difference $(y-x)$	Before injection	After injection	Difference $(y-x)$	Before injection	After injection	Difference $(y-x)$	
1	1		1	1		1	1		
2	2		2	2		2	2		
3	3		3	3		3	3		
Initial temp. (x)	4		Initial temp. (x)	4		Initial temp. (x)	4		
	5			5			5		
	6			6			6		
	Max. temp.(y)			Max. temp.(y)			Max. temp.(y)		

Experiment 13

OBJECT

To carry out test for pyrogen IP edition 1996 (main test).

Preparation of sample

Dissolve the substance being examined in or diluted with pyrogen free saline solution or other solution prescribed in the monograph. Warm the liquid being examined to approximately 38.5° C before injecting.

Dose

The volume of injection is not less than 0.5 ml per kg and not more 10 ml per kg of body weight.

Procedure

Take three selected rabbits of the previous experiments. Record the temperature of each animal at the interval of not more than 30 minutes, beginning at least 90 minutes before the injection of the solution being examined and continuing for three hours after the injection. Not more than 90 minutes immediately preceding the injection of the test dose, record the Initial temperature of each rabbit, which is the mean of two temperature recorded for that rabbit at an interval of 30 minutes in 40 minutes period. Rabbits showing a temperature variation greater than 0.2° C between two successive readings in the determination of "Initial temperature", should not be used for the test. In any one group of the test animal, use only those animals whose "initial temperatures" do not vary by more than 1° C from each other and do not use any rabbit having a temperature higher than 39.8° C and lower than 38° C.

Inject the solution being examined slowly in to the marginal vein of the ear of each rabbit over a period not exceeding four minute unless otherwise prescribed in the monograph. Record the temperature of the each rabbit at half hourly intervals for three hours after the injection. The difference between "initial temperature" and the maximum temperature which is the highest temperature recorded for a rabbit is taken to be its response. When this difference is negative the result is considered as a zero response.

Interpretation

If the sum of responses of the group of three rabbits does not exceed 1.4° C and if the response of any individual rabbit is less than 0.6° C, the preparation being examined passes the test. If the response of any rabbit is 0.6° C or more, or if the sum of the responses of the three rabbits exceeds 1.4° C, continue the test using five other rabbits. If not more than three of the eight rabbits show individual responses of 0.6° C or more, and if the sum of responses of group of eight rabbits does not exceed 3.7° C, the preparation being examined passes the test.

Result

The sample of the test—Passed/failed the test.

Drug	Trade name	Name of company
Chlorpromazine	Megatil injection	INTAS
Chlorpromazine	Chlorpromazine injection	NICHOLAS

Experiment 14

OBJECT

To study the taming effect of chlorpromazine in mice/rats.

Requirements

Cooke's pole climbing apparatus, syringes, rats, etc.

Chemicals

Saline solution, chlorpromazine–4 mg per kg body wt., etc.

Principle

Chlorpromazine is antipsychotic drug belongs to phenothiazine group. It has got therapeutic application in treatment of schizophrenia and aggressiveness. Chlorpromazine produces a variety of actions on CNS. It blocks the conditional avoidance response in animals, also produces sedation and prolong sleeping time of barbiturates. This action of chlorpromazine is studied on rats using pole climbing apparatus.

This apparatus has an experimental chamber with floor grid enclosure. The enclosure has a sliding door of acrylic perfex plastic for viewing of the electronic controls which provide both types of stimuli, i.e. audible and electrical. The pole is of two portions and is placed in the lid on the top of the chamber. The smaller portion works as a handle and the longer one serves as a pole which hangs in side the chamber. In front has arrangement for sliding door. Upper lid will allow a animal to be introduced in to or removed from the chamber. A sliding tray is provided beneath the floor grid which can be pulled out for cleaning.

The rat feels shock when he moves at any place at the bottom of the apparatus. The pole is the only safe place for rat to avoid shock. The apparatus is designed as such that it gives danger signal such as buzzer sound before giving shock. The rat is trained for the above things. By hearing only the sound of buzzer if the rat climbs up on the pole to protect himself from the shock, the training is considered complete. This is called conditional avoidance response. Chlorpromazine selectively blocks such responses but not the non-conditional response (direst response to electric shock).

Procedure

Take two healthy rats of identical sex and weigh. Both of them are trained to climb up on the pole to escape from electric shock. They are also trained to avoid electric shock by responding quickly to buzzer sound. Inject one ml saline solution to first rat intraperitoneally and put in pole climbing chamber and observe the response by giving buzzer sound followed by shock. Latter on the same rat (saline treated) is subjected to direct electric shock and note the response. To another rat inject specific dose of chlorpromazine (4 mg per kg) intraperitoneally and repeat the same procedure as above and note the response.

Result

Chlorpromazine treated rat does not show response to buzzer sound since the drug selectively blocks the conditional avoidance response where as the saline treated rat shows both the responses, i.e. conditional avoidance (to climb on pole by hearing buzzer sound followed by shock) and unconditional avoidance (to climb on the pole in response to direct shock.

Experiment 15

OBJECT

To study the effect of diphenyl-hydramine in experimentally produced asthma in guinea pigs.

Requirements

Histamine chamber, guinea pigs, syringes, etc.

Chemicals

Histamine diphosphate 5%.
Diphenyl hydramine hydrochloride 2.5 mg per kg.

Principle

Histamine is beta imidazole ethylamine. It is synthesized from aminoacid histadine. It under goes decarboxylation to form histamine. It is bound to acid group like carboxyl, thiol and phosphate of the cellular proteins. It acts through two receptors-H1 and H2. H1 receptors are present in intestine, bronchi, uterus, etc. and on stimulation produce contraction of smooth muscles of these tissues. Stimulation of H2 receptors produce dilatation of blood vessels, increase in gastric acid secretion.

Diphenyl-hydramine is a H1 receptor antagonist (antihistaminics) belongs to ethanolamines class. It blocks histamine induced allergy, anaphylaxis, triple response, hypotension, headache and contraction of smooth muscles. It has sedative action also. For in vivo testing of histamine and antihistaminics guinea pig is used. It is very sensitive to histamine and fatal asthma is readily produced in this animal when exposed to histamine aerosol.

Procedure

Select two healthy guinea pigs of either sex weighing between 250–300 gm and withhold food from animal over night. Inject saline solution to one guinea pig intraperitoneally and dyphenyl hydramine hydrochloride to another one. After one an hour, place the animal in histamine chamber, one in each compartment. Spray the histamine diphosphate aerosol from a nebuliser in both the compartments. Observe the both animals for signs of broncho-spasm, cessation of breathing, asphyxial convulsions. Note time to on set of these symptoms and compare the results obtained in two guinea pigs.

Result

The saline treated guinea pig shows brochospasm, cessation of breathing and head drop where as diphenyl hydramine treated guinea pig does not show any such symptoms. It proves the antihistaminic action of diphenyl hydramine.

Observation table

S. No.	Rat no	Reaction time in seconds		
		Minutes after injection of morphine		
		15 minutes	30 minutes	60 minutes
1.	Rat No–1 (saline treated)	....	....	....
2.	Rat No–2 (morphine treated)	....	....	....

Note

More reaction time in case of rat no–2 proves the analgesic activity of morphine.

Market preparation

Drug	Trade name	Company name
Morphine	Morphine	Alembic
Pentazocine	Fortwin	Ranbaxy

Experiment 16

OBJECT

To demonstrate the operation of analgesiometer or to study the analgesic activity of drugs by anagesiometer.

Requirement

Analgesiometer.

Chemicals

Saline, morphine—150 mg per kg, etc.

Principle

Analgesics are drugs which relieve from pain. Analgesic is classified as narcotic and non-narcotic analgesic. Non-narcotic analgesics interfere with relay of pain impulses at the thalamic levels. They possess anti-inflammatory and antipyretic action also. Experimental pain can be produce chemically, mechanically, electrically and thermally. Analgesic activity of narcotic can be evaluated effectively by analgesiometer. The instrument has a heated nichrome wire for producing pain in the rat's tail. The temperature of the wire is kept constant. There is arrangement for circulating water at room temperature around the rat's tail and nichrome wire to keep the environment nearly cool. It is based on the reaction of the rat to heat stimulus applied to the tail. The instrument is provided with digital readout and reset arrangement to note the reaction time in seconds and on/off switches.

Procedure

Select two healthy rats of either sex. The control rat is treated with saline solution and the test rat is injected morphine (150 mg per kg) subcutaneously. Note the reaction time for the both rats after half hour and one hour of injection. Prolongation of reaction is the indicative of the analgesic activity of morphine.

Reaction time

After placing the rat in rat retaining box. Its tail is placed over the wire. When the rat becomes quiet and stable in this position, the circuit is completed in anagesiometer. Note the time interval in seconds by digital readout of analgesiometer as rat withdraws its tail with a sudden and characteristics flick. This is called reaction time.

Observation table

Animal No.	Drug	Dose	Activity after injection			
			15 minutes	*30 minutes*	*45 minutes*	*60 minutes*
1.	Saline solution	1 ml	....	....	....	....
2.	Diazepam	4 mg per kg	....	....	....	....
3.	Leptazole	80 mg per kg	....	....	....	....

Experiment 17

OBJECT

To study the operation of photoactometer (activity cage).

Requirement

Photoactometer activity cage, rats or mice.

Chemicals

Leptazole, strychnine, phenobarbitone, diazepam, etc.

Principle

CNS stimulant drugs increase the activity of animal where as CNS depressant drugs decrease the activity of the animals. Leptazole stimulates cortex, respiratory centre and spinal cord. CNS depressant drugs (barbiturates, benzodiazepines) produce drowsiness, sedation, hypnosis and loss of consciousness. Thus they reduce the activity of animals.

Thus digital photoactometer is used to study the effect of drugs acting on CNS with spontaneous ambulatory activities of small animals such as rats and mice. Photoactometer consists of highly sensitive solid state light receivers and transmitters. It is provided with a activity cage of wall $30 \times 30 \times 30$ cm^3 in dimensions with a wire mesh floor. Six pairs of light transmitters and receivers are so placed around the outer periphery of activity cage that they form a mesh of beam in shape of square. The interrupted light signals are further converted into electrical ones through a compact solid state circuitry and the activity is recorded on a bright high speed digital counter for display. It also consists of zero reset and a sliding tray at the bottom to clean the excreta of the animal.

Procedure

Select three rats of either sex with approximate identical weight. One rat is treated intraperitoneally with saline solution. Inject the diazepam (4 mg per kg body weight) intraperitoneally to second rat and leptazole (80 mg per kg body weight) to third one. Record the activity of all three rats for specific time.

Result

The saline treated rat shows normal activity. Leptazole is a CNS stimulant drug, produces more activity than that of normal where as diazepam is CNS depressant drug, produces less activity than that of normal.

Experiment 18

OBJECT

Experiment 19

OBJECT

Experiment 20

OBJECT

Viva Voce

Q1. What is lever?

Ans. It is a recording device used in experimental pharmacology for magnifying the events that occur in the tissue. It has got a short and a long arm. The writing point is attached at the tip of the long arm of the lever.

Q2. Enlist the different types of levers.

Ans. 1. Simple lever
2. Frontal writing lever
3. Sterlings heart lever
4. Universal lever
5. Gimbal lever

Q3. Write important characteristics of good lever.

Ans. 1. It should be as light as possible to avoid wastage of energy.
2. Rotation across the fulcrum should be frictionless.
3. Lever should be made up of rigid material like aluminium or stainless steel.
4. Load must be as close to the fulcrum as possible.

Q4. Why fixing of smoked paper is essential?

Ans. Fixing of smoked paper is essential to make the record permanent.

Q5. How fixing of smoked paper is carried out?

Ans. Make a 5% solution of resin (shellac or colophony) in sprit. The smoked paper is dipped in above prepared reginous solution. It is allowed to drain and dry. The operation should be carried out in dust free environment.

Q6. Define agonist.

Ans. It is a substance which elicits response (contraction of muscle).

Q7. Define antagonist.

Ans. It is a substance which counteracts the response of agonist, i.e. prevents contractions of muscle.

Q8. What is minimum effective dose?

Ans. It is the concentration of a substance which elicits a just measurable response.

Q9. Define ED 50 (median effective dose).

Ans. It is dose which elicits 50% of maximum possible response.

Q10. What is sub-maximal dose and maximum dose?

Ans. Sub-maximal dose—A dose of substance which produces a response just below the maximum possible response.

Maximum dose—It is a dose of substance which produces maximum response. Just above this dose, there is no increase of response of a substance being examined.

Q11. What is physiological salt solution?

Ans. The solution used in organ bath, provides nutrition to isolated tissue is termed as physiological salt solution.

Q12. Write the role of ions and glucose in the perfusion fluid.

Ans. Sodium chloride—It provides sodium ions which maintain isotonicity, excitability and contractility of the preparation.

Potassium chloride—It provides potassium ions which is essential for relaxation of muscle . It also has some catalytic action for sodium ions.

Calcium chloride—It provides calcium ions which maintain contractility of the preparation. In absence of calcium ions in the perfusion fluid, isolated preparation fails to contract vigorously. Thus the actions of K^+ and Ca^{++} ions are opposing to each other.

Sodium or potassium dihydrogen phosphate— It acts as a buffer.

Glucose—It provides nutrition.

Magnesium chloride or sulphate—They stabilize the preparation and hence to reduce the spontaneous activity.

Q13. Write uses of the following physiological solutions

Frog ringer, tyrode, Krebs, dejalon and ringer lock's solution.

Ans. Frog ringer—It is used for tissue of frog like heart, rectus abdominis muscle and others.

Ringer lock's—It is used for mammalian cardiac and for smooth muscle experiments.

Tyrode—It is used for guinea pig ileum, rat ileum, rabbit ileum, etc. where spontaneous motility is not desired.

Dejalon—It is used for rat uterus.

Krebs—It is used for rat fundus strip, vas-deferens, etc.

Q14. Write the advantage of using frontal writing lever.

Ans. It gives a record with a uniform friction and the writing point falls vertically against the paper. The traces thus obtained are linear.

Q15. What is the purpose of aeration?

Ans. (a) To provide oxygen to the preparation.

(b) To help in uniform distribution of drugs.

Q16. What is euthanasia?

Ans. Painless killing of an animal is called euthanasia.

Q17. What is pithing of frog?

Ans. Destruction of brain and spinal cord by stunning (sudden hammering of head of frog against hard material like edge of table), than piercing a needle through depression in to the skull and vertebral column respectively.

Q18. Why does the temperature of the inner organ bath not maintain in case of amphibian tissue (frog).

Ans. The frog is poikilothermic animal. So temperature of inner organ bath containing the physiological solution and isolated tissue is not maintained.

Q19. In case of mammalian tissue how and why the temperature of inner organ bath containing the physiological solution and isolated tissue is maintained?

Ans. The mammals are warm blooded animal so temperature is maintained at 37° C by filling the outer bath with warm water or by using thermostat.

Q20. Enlist commonly used general anaesthetics to produce unconsiousness to experimental animals.

Ans.

Drug	Concentration	Dose per kg	Route
Urethane	25%	1.5 gm	IV
Pentobarbitone	6%	25 mg	IP/IV
Thiopentone sodium	2.5%	12-26 mg	IV

IV- Intravenous

IP- Intraperitoneal

Q21. Write the experimental uses of rabbit as animal in pharmacology.

Ans. This animal is widely used for study of pyrogen testing, hypoglycemic drug, tetratogens and serological works. Rabbit also helps in study of drugs effecting reproductive system.

Q22. Write the utility of guinea pig in experimental pharmacology.

Ans. It is highly sensitive to histamine so this animal is used for evaluation of antihistaminic drug. It is also used for study of tuberculosis. The isolated tissue of guinea pig is useful for bioassay of histamine and acetylcholine.

Q23. Write some peculiarities of rats.

Ans. Rat does not possess vomiting center, tonsil or a gall bladder.

Q24. Why should physiological salt solution be prepared freshly?

Ans. Because it is good media for growth of microorganism. After removing the glucose and calcium chloride, it should be preserve in refrigerator. Glucose and calcium chloride should be added at the time of experiment.

Q25. Define receptor.

Ans. It is hypothetical specific cellular components with which drugs combine chemically to evolve the biological response.

Q26. Write the name of receptor found in parasympathomimetics.

Ans. Muscarinic receptor and nicotinic receptor.

Q27. Write pharmacological actions of acetylcholine.

Ans. 1. It decreases the force and frequency of heart muscle.
2. It causes contraction of smooth muscle.
3. It causes miosis of eye (constriction of pupil).
4. It also causes contraction of skeletal muscle.

Q28. What type of receptor is found is rectus abdominis muscle of frog?

Ans. Nicotinic receptor.

Q29. Write the action of adrenaline on heart.

Ans. Adrenaline increases heart rate, force of contraction, cardiac out put and systolic blood pressure.

Q30. Write therapeutic uses of adrenaline.

Ans. Bronchial asthma, anaphylactic shock, local haemostatic and cardiac syncope.

Q31. Parasympatholytics and sympathomimetics produce mydriasis. What is difference between them?

Ans.

Parasympatholytics	*Sympathomimetics*
1. They cause mydriasis by action of circular muscle.	1. They cause mydriasis by action of radial muscle.
2. They cause cycloplegia.	2. They do not cause.

Q32. What is cycloplegia?

Ans. The loss of accommodation is called cycloplegia.

Q33. Write the action of histamine. Why it was sprayed as aerosol on guinea pig?

Ans Guinea pig is very sensitive to histamine action. It causes marked contraction of the bronchial musculature giving rise to asthma and asphyxia (decrease in gaseous exchange). The oedematous swelling of bronchioles is associated with bronchial asthma .

Q34. Write the name of histamine receptors.

Ans. 1. H_1 receptor–It causes allergy, triple response, headache and contraction of smooth muscles.
2. H_2 receptor–It has role in gastric acid secretion.

Q35. Write the therapeutic uses of diphenyl hydramine.

Ans. Allergy, anaphylactic shock, triple response, motion sickness and as sedative.

Q36. Enlist the name of anticonvulsants.

Ans. Phenyltoin, phenobarbitone, trimethadione, Phensuximide, carbazepine and sodium valproate.

Q37. Define epilepsy.

Ans. Epilepsy is chronic CNS disorder characterized by brief episodes of seizures convulsion and loss of consciousness.

Q38. Define convulsion.

Ans. Violent spasmodic contraction of skeletal muscle is called convulsion.

Q39. Classify epilepsy.

Ans. (1) Focal epilepsy
(2) Temporal epilepsy

(3) Grand–mal epilepsy

(4) Petit-mal epilepsy

Q40. Enlist the name of convulsing agents.

Ans. The most of the analeptics in large doses act as convulgants, e.g.. Picrotoxin, nikethamide, leptazole, strychnine, etc.

Q41. Write therapeutic uses of leptazole.

Ans. As cardiorespiratory stimulant and schizophrenia.

Q42. What is schizophrenia?

Ans. It is a type of psychiatric disorder characterized by disturb thinking, delusion and auditory hallucination.

Q43. Write therapeutic uses of chlorpromazine.

Ans. Schizophrenia, anti emetic and destructive behaviour in children.

Q44. Write the effects of strychnine in frog.

Ans. Strychnine produces tonic type of convulsions, lock jaw and bending of body.

Q45. Write the effect of digitalis on heart.

Ans. It increases the force of myocardial heart muscle contraction and increases the cardiac output. When digitalis is given to the patient of CCF, there is a increase in force of contraction of the heart and hence there is increases in cardiac output. The end systole volume is decreased, causing decrease in size of the heart. It increases the energy utilization for contraction of heart muscle.

Q46. Write therapeutic uses of digitalis.

Ans. Congestive cardiac failure, atrial flutter, atrial fibrillation and paroxysmal atrial tachycardia.

Q47. Who did discover digitalis?

Ans. William Withering discovered digitalis in 1776.

Q48. Write application of photo-actometer.

Ans. It is used to study the effect of drugs acting on CNS with spontaneous ambulatory activities of small animals such as rats or mice.

Q49. Write the application of histamine chamber.

Ans. Histamine chamber is used to evaluate the antihistaminic action of drugs like diphenyl hydramine, promethazine, etc.

Q50. Write the application of electroconvulsometer.

Ans. It is used to study the effect of anticonvulsant or antiepileptic drugs. In this apparatus convulsion is produced in animals like rats or mice by electrically induced shock. Phenyltoin prevents tonic convulsions produced by maximum electric shock.